RAISE YOUR VIBRATION
WITH NUTRITION & FASTING

D1568818

Raise Your Vibration with Nutrition & Fasting

Nogah Lord

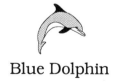

Blue Dolphin

Copyright © 1991 Nogah Lord
All rights reserved.

Illustrations: Eran Elkayam & Gali Nahar

Published by Blue Dolphin Publishing, Inc.
P.O. Box 1908, Nevada City, CA 95959

ISBN: 0-931892-68-6

Library of Congress Cataloging-in-Publication Data

Lord, Nogah, 1942–
    Raise your vibration with nutrition & fasting /
    Nogah Lord.
        p.   cm.
    Includes bibliographical references.
    ISBN 0-931892-68-6 : $8.95
    1. Nutrition. 2. Fasting. 3. Vegetarianism.
    I. Title.
    RA784.L67 1991
    613.7—dc20   91-27781
                              CIP

Printed on recycled paper
in the United States of America by
Blue Dolphin Press, Inc., Grass Valley, California

10   9   8   7   6   5   4   3

Dear Reader,

This book is a practical guide for natural living. It offers information about health from my own personal experience. It is not intended to serve as a substitute for examination, diagnosis and treatment by certified health professionals. Each person is responsible for the results s/he receives.

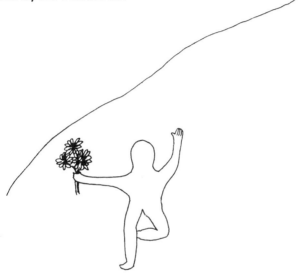

I want to thank all the friends who assisted in preparing this book, especially Gloria Bat-El for her help with the layout and typing of the original. Thanks also to Martha Corley and Donald Seaman for their encouragement and editing suggestions.

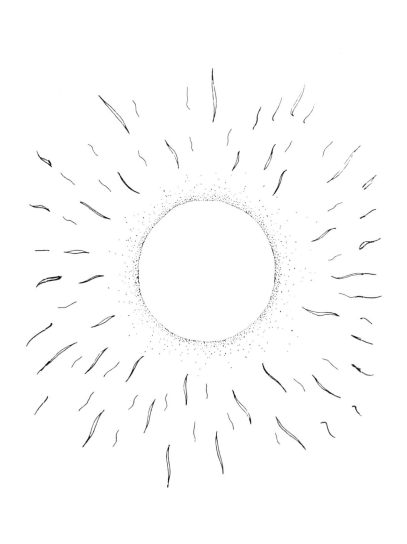

Table of Contents

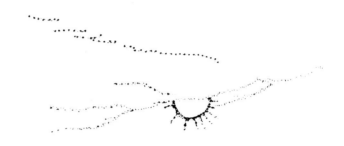
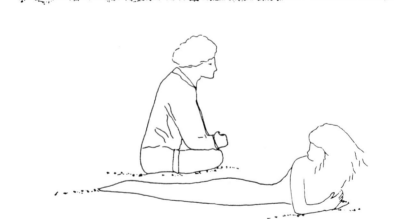

Foreword

IN 1964, ABOUT TWO YEARS AFTER I started dancing professionally, I had my first enlightenment. I realized that God was in me! And therefore in everyone! This was not only an intellectual realization; it was something I experienced in my whole being. From that moment on, I was never the same. In the following months, I could hardly sleep or eat. I was filled with energy, love and joy. I started writing and drawing the impressions I was receiving about reality. At that time I didn't understand what had happened or why it happened. It took me about twenty years to begin to understand.

In this book, I share some of my life experiences and fundamental understandings.

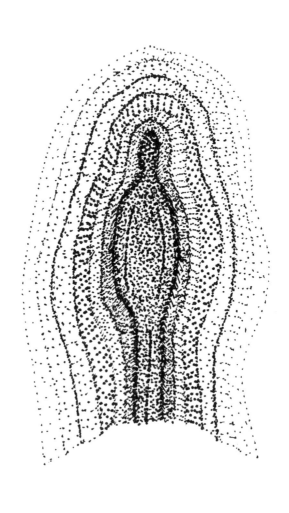

Understanding
Ourselves

EVERYTHING IS MADE UP OF ENERGY. The main difference among various forms of life is their frequency of vibration. The more highly evolved the life form, the higher its frequency of vibration. The same is also true regarding human beings. The more highly evolved a human being is, the higher his vibrations. Aging and sickness are a sign of a slowing down of vibrations. A healthy youth will vibrate at a higher rate than an unhealthy youth.

In ancient times, the more evolved members of a community were healers. Their mere presence had a healing effect. Because of their higher vibrations, they were able to raise the vibrations of those around them and those who needed to be healed. In fact, throughout recorded history we find that all saints were healers. So, it stands to reason that healthy and superhuman beings vibrate at a higher rate than unhealthy, ordinary humans.

Our physical body is an exact replica of our mental body. It is one of seven bodies we can occupy. Each of the seven bodies surrounds our physical form and vibrates at a different frequency. Most of us function in three bodies only: the physical, mental and emotional bodies.

Only those who consciously begin to control the three bodies go on to develop their fourth body and eventually all seven. To accomplish this, one needs a teacher, someone who has gained experience in this endeavor. Anyone can be your teacher if that person vibrates at a higher level than you do.

Your body is your airplane. In it you travel through life. It has the ability to fly but most people utilize it only on the ground. A teacher is someone who can soar into the air and therefore can see far more than you. Having a teacher saves time and energy and enables you to accomplish much more. Eventually you may raise your vibration and learn to fly as well. Then you will personally comprehend things that are beyond your grasp right now.

To fly one needs energy. In the following chapters we will discuss some of the ways energy is acquired.

Acquiring Energy

TO RAISE YOUR VIBRATION you need energy. But most of the energy you receive is spent solely in maintaining your physical body. So you need to start learning how to conserve what you have and how to create more.

Energy comes via food, sleep, and performance of one's duty. And there are laws which govern these functions.

Nourishment should be derived from real, fresh, uncontaminated foods. The right amount should be consumed in the right way, and at the right time of day. Sleep should also occur at the right time, in the right way and in the right amount.

Performing your duties means fulfilling your obligations—first toward yourself, then toward your family, your country, your world and your Creator.

Performing your duties means living according to right and true principles, living according to your conscience, **doing** what you think is right and **not doing** what you think is wrong.

Living a disciplined life and going against your automatic, mechanical behavior provides tremendous energy that you cannot receive otherwise.

Energy is lost through improper use of body, mind and spirit.

Improper use of the body:

- Disturbed sleep or too much sleep.
- Eating too much or the wrong foods.
- Suppression of sex or too much of it.
- Too much talking about the wrong things.
- Not enough physical exercise or too much.

Improper use of the mind:

- Being dishonest.
- Brooding over the past.
- Worrying about the future.
- Not spending enough time in contemplation.
- Dwelling in negativity and suppressing feelings.

Improper use of the spirit:

- Ignoring your conscience.
- Living in fear instead of love.
- Being concerned only for yourself.
- Not living according to right and true principles.
- Not setting aside times for silence and meditation.

We accumulate energy by leading disciplined lives and organizing our lives in such a way that our physical, mental and emotional bodies are balanced and our spiritual needs are met.

In the next chapter there is a description of how I unintentionally raised my vibration without proper preparation. In the following chapters I will discuss how you can prepare your body and mind for higher rates of vibrations.

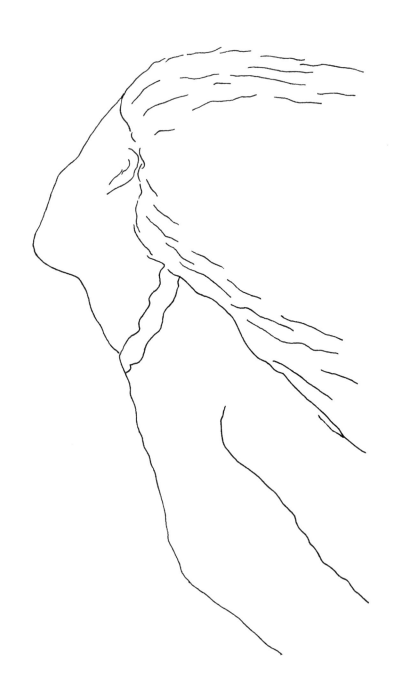

How I Raised My Vibration

W HEN I LEFT ISRAEL for America at age 13, I was in perfect health. My hair was lustrous, my skin smooth and radiant, my teeth were white with no cavities. I was calm, confident and cheerful. I had been raised in an extremely healthy environment on a kibbutz. Our diet consisted of organic fruits and vegetables with very little meat and almost no sweets— along with daily exercise in the fresh air.

After six years of living on the typical American diet with fatty meats, fried foods, and all kinds of sweets, I started dancing professionally. Although I appeared strong and vital, actually my health was deteriorating. As a professional dancer, I worked six nights a week, went to bed between 4:30 and 6:00 A.M., and was up at 8:00 or 9:00 A.M., sleeping between two and four hours out of 24 and eating once a day. I spent most of my time walking, dancing, writing and drawing. I did very little talking and only had sex on rare occasions.

Every night while dancing I experienced altered states of consciousness. I lost contact with ordinary reality perceived through the five senses. I was functioning in a different reality and in an altered time frame.

Physically, I experienced short electric shocks along my spine. Mentally, my mind became quieter. Emotionally, I felt love and joy far beyond anything experienced in my ordinary state of consciousness.

During my performances I was so detached from my physical body that I could hardly hear or see what went on around me. Even my physical appearance changed, which can clearly be seen in photos taken during that time. But I also was experiencing a nagging pain in my lower back which steadily got worse.

Only when I was actually dancing and got into one of those trance states was I free of pain.

I did not understand what state I was in. All I knew was that I wanted to experience more of it. I couldn't wait to go to work every night and dance.

Life was filled with new meanings. It was both exciting and a mystery. I saw life as a movie with myself and everyone else as actors in it. I couldn't wait to experience the next scenes, always expecting new and wonderful things to happen. But all around me people were very negative. To me life was obviously a movie and the actors had to know the outcome. Why were they taking themselves so seriously, and why were they so unkind to one another?

I found such inner contentment that I no longer had the need for approval or to control anything or anyone. When someone was negative, I just moved out of the way. I was becoming happier and more content and felt as good being with myself as being with others. With so much love inside, there was no need to look for it elsewhere.

Without realizing it, everything I was doing was elevating my vibration even more. But because I was physically, mentally and emotionally unprepared, the energy being raised along my spine was getting trapped half-way up. As a result there was a war inside my body. The upper portion above my waist was being pulled up while the bottom portion below my waist was being pulled down. At times the pain was so severe that I could hardly speak or breathe.

In January of 1972, I became paralyzed. In this state—flat on my back in terrible pain, unable to move any part of my body except my hands—I began my great spiritual journey. I read books on healing, natural health and spiritual development, became a vegetarian, stopped smoking, drinking and taking medications, and started meditating twice a day. I met with other spiritual aspirants and their teachers.

Although my physical activity was very limited, my mental activity was on the rise. I received answers to many of my questions and began a process of building up my physical and mental health, letting go of resentments and fears and learning to communicate my true feelings. I forgave my parents and friends for wrongs I believed they had committed and took responsibility for what happened in my life.

I began to erase negative behavior patterns by daily writing positive affirmations and associating only with people who were supportive and loving.

As my physical and mental health improved, I began having conscious out-of-body experiences which followed a speeding up of energy and a buzzing sound, similar to the sensation felt when an airplane is about to take off. Occasionally during fasts I could see the human aura in color and even saw spiritual beings around certain people. I did not find others with whom I could share these experiences, and those I found said they had similar experiences only under the influence of drugs.

After many years of observation and experimentation I came to the conclusion that you can raise your vibration and heighten perception if you do the following:

- Eat less.
- Talk less.
- Sleep less.
- Breathe more.
- Exercise more.
- Meditate more.
- Bless everyone.
- Be absolutely truthful.
- Let go of all resentments.

We are electric beings. At present we vibrate at a particular rate and, according to that rate, our levels of understanding and intelligence are determined. To expand understanding and heighten our intelligence we need to receive more energy into our systems. For this we need to make preparations. The vehicle must be operating in perfect order and be in top physical condition. The mind and emotions must be balanced.

In the following chapters you can learn how to prepare yourself.

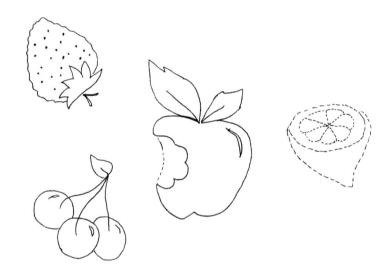

Right Nutrition

W E EAT IN ORDER TO RECEIVE ENERGY. Energy comes from the sun, the air, the water, and the earth. By going directly to the earth for our food, we not only conserve energy used for digestion and assimilation, but also receive a finer energy which can be used for higher purposes. The more natural the food, the more energy it has. Unfortunately, most of us are in the habit of eating the wrong things for the wrong reasons. For example, the energy received from the animals we eat is indirect. The animal received its energy from the food of the earth. In order to digest unnatural food, processed or cooked food, our body needs to slow down and use more energy to assimilate it.

The position of the sun greatly influences our digestion. It is easier to digest food eaten in the daytime than at night. The ideal breakfast time is at least two hours past sunrise and after some physical activity. Dinner should be light and at least two hours before sunset. Lunch should be your heaviest meal. Whenever possible eat the heavier meals early in the day and the lighter meals later in the day. Don't go to bed with a full stomach.

As your body becomes more balanced you will find yourself automatically eating the right things at the right time. It takes between seven and forty days to retrain and return the body to correct eating habits. *Fasting is a great aid in this endeavor.* Eventually, you will eat only when and what is necessary to maintain your body.

The following foods are listed according to how much energy they give and the time it takes for digestion and assimilation. The more real, alive, and unprocessed the food, the more energy it gives and the less energy it takes to assimilate it.

Food List from the Lightest to the Heaviest

1. Pure water
2. Fresh fruit
3. Sprouts and live vegetables
4. Sesame, sunflower, pumpkin seeds and nuts (raw)
5. Dried fruit

6. Steamed or cooked vegetables
*7. Natural brown rice
8. Wheat, legumes, cereals
9. Whole wheat crackers, breads, biscuits
10. Soy products
11. Dairy products

12. Eggs
13. Fish
14. Poultry
15. Lamb, beef
16. Pork

*Brown rice is a balanced food that can be eaten at every meal. Great for those on a transition diet. Has a calming effect.

The list is divided into three types of food:

From 1 to 5 — Light food, easy to digest, full of water. More suitable for the spiritually evolved and for those living closer to nature.

From 6 to 11 — Cooked and processed food, heavier to digest, but suitable for the average human being especially those who live in cities.

From 12 to 16 — Heavy food, difficult to digest, and suitable for those addicted to food. It is the type of food that sticks to the walls of the colon, causes constipation, thickens the blood and causes swelling in the veins, arteries and muscles. This food is eaten out of ignorance and habit.

Example of a Day's Menu

Upon waking — Pure water with or without lemon juice or honey. Herbal tea or fresh juice from fruits or sprouts which can be mixed with pure water. Especially beneficial is wheat grass juice.

Breakfast — Two hours or more after sunrise and after meditation and exercise.

Ripe fruit in season or soaked dried fruit (prunes, figs, raisins) with raw nuts. Or fruit mixed in blender with a teaspoon of tahini.*

Lunch — Vegetable salad with all types of sprouts and two baked potatoes. Or natural brown rice with steamed vegetables and beans. Or a thick soup with whole wheat bread; spread with either sesame tahini or margarine from sunflower seeds or soy.

Dinner — Before sunset.

Fresh vegetables with natural yogurt or cheese. Or tofu with nuts and seeds. Or fruit salad with nuts and a dressing from tahini diluted with water and honey.

*Tahini — Butter made from ground sesame seeds. Sesame seeds are very tasty and rich in vitamins, minerals, and protein. They contain an abundance of calcium.

In between meals — fruit or vegetable juices and herbal teas.

Tasty juice — 10 soaked dates and 20 peeled almonds with or without two bananas, one apple or one pear mixed with pure water; puree in blender.

- Eat fresh food before cooked food.
- Do not eat fruits and vegetables in the same meal. Let at least two hours pass between eating fruits and vegetables.
- Do not eat before bed. If hungry, drink herb tea or juice from one fruit only.

Items harmful to the body — white flour, white sugar, salt, coffee, preservatives, food coloring, alcohol, nicotine, synthetic medicine and drugs.

To return to the right way of eating may look simple, but it is not always easy. Both the body and mind have become addicted to many bad habits for many years. So you must be patient with yourself as you begin to add some good eating habits and start to eliminate the bad ones.

There is no doubt that a change in eating habits can be a challenging and interesting adventure. You will be happy to discover that you spend less time, energy and money by living on the right foods.

The foods you eat have an effect on you. But your thoughts about what you are eating affect you more than the food itself. Your thoughts are more powerful than your body and your senses. So, no matter what you eat, eat it after blessing it and affirming that the body will take what it needs and reject what is harmful to it. If you find difficulty in giving up certain foods, why not try Dr. West's way? Eat what you think is right six days a week; on the seventh day, eat whatever you desire.

After realizing the harmful effects animal foods can have on the body, Dr. West and his wife switched to a pure vegetarian diet: eliminating all dairy and all products made with white sugar as well. Their dilemma was how to break the news to their seven children. They decided to prepare a variety of nutritious and attractive meals each day. But every Sunday they took the children to their favorite restaurant where they could eat anything they wanted—meat, cheese, and even ice cream and cake.

This program went on for a few weeks and then slowly each of the children declined to go on their Sunday spree. They said that they preferred the food at home. Within a few months, all seven children had chosen to become vegetarians.

For me, changing from meat-eating to vegetarianism was a gradual process. At first, I gave up only beef and sugar, thinking it would only be until I got well. But then I found myself unable to consume even chicken. Later on the desire for fish fell away as well.

Then I decided to give up dairy and all flour products. It was a decision my body was not really ready for, so I went through withdrawal symptoms. My cravings for cheese and bread were so strong that I often gave in and "cheated." I learned from past experience not to judge myself too harshly because that only prompted me to cheat more. I got back to my discipline as soon as the cravings subsided. Throughout this transition my original decision to eliminate bread and cheese never changed.

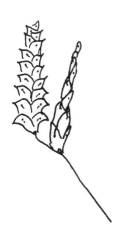

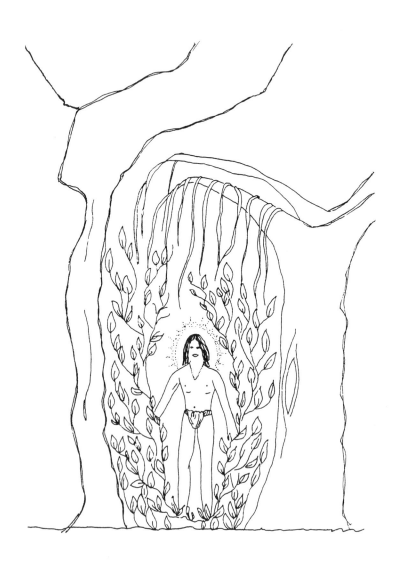

Benefits of Becoming a Vegetarian

Within two years on the vegetarian diet I noticed the following:

- I could sit still and silently for hours.
- There were no new cavities in my teeth.
- My hair grew thick again and was silky and shiny.
- My breathing became deeper and easier.
- I slept quietly without tossing and awakened early, feeling refreshed and clear no matter what time I went to bed.
- My taste buds became sharper and so did my senses of sight, smell, touch and hearing.
- No more colds every winter.

- I became more conscious of my body's needs and its overall condition. I received very clear indications of what to eat and when to stop.
- In winter I tolerated the cold and in summer the heat. When the weather changed abruptly I didn't suffer.
- I was attracted only to healthy, nutritious food and was repelled by junk food.
- My posture became straight while sitting, standing or walking.
- I stopped having accidents and injuring my body, such as:
  —Biting my tongue while eating.
  —Scratching myself with my nails.
  —Burning myself while ironing or cooking.
  —Cutting myself.
  —Falling down often.
- I developed many new talents. My intuition and instincts became keener.
- My memory improved and so did my ability to concentrate.

You have read only a few of the benefits I received as a result of changing my eating habits

and meditating regularl̖
achievements every day. Yc
health and harmony no matt
dition. All that is required is a
along with *consistency* and aι
goal. Once you start, you will m
will guide and support you. I staɪ   ̖ut
very soon received help and encoι   ̖cment. I
am now truly content and happy. You can be,
too.

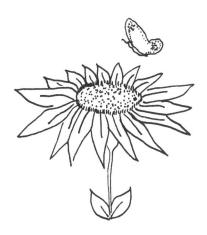

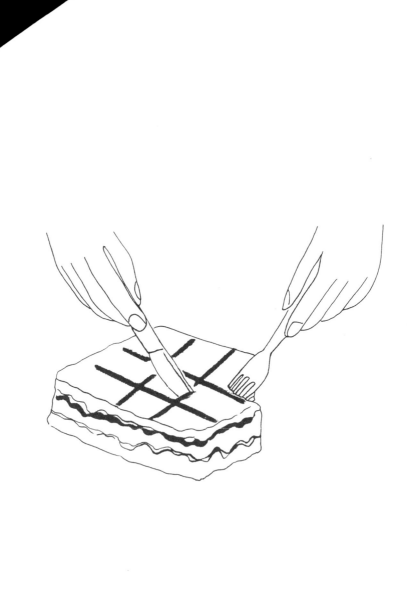

Obstacles on the Way

WHETHER YOU CHANGE YOUR DIET from meat-eating to vegetarianism, from cooked food to consuming only raw food, or from eating your food to drinking it, you may encounter some obstacles.

Upon being introduced to a new way of life—one you believe will improve your condition—you become hopeful and excited. This gives you the incentive to make a commitment to a program of self-renewal and rehabilitation. At the start of the program you are proud for having taken the first steps. Then you look for approval and support from your family and friends, which may or may not be forthcoming. If you do not get enough support, you may become less enthusiastic. In this condition you continue on your path. If you feel you are not making progress, you may not have the will to continue. If you *do* see progress, you may go on with your discipline.

Now you may encounter the next obstacle. As your body goes through its cleansing process and as the memories of your past eating habits start to play through your mind, you will start to experience strong cravings for the very items that you are trying to avoid. When this happens, there are several different ways to deal with the problem. One approach is to ignore it, knowing it is a temporary situation. (In fact the cravings are strongest when the body is getting rid of residues through the blood.) The other approach is to take a little of the food that you crave and allow yourself to enjoy it, without judging yourself for doing it. Remember, changing yourself takes time and perseverance.

It is important to have enough knowledge about what you are attempting and sufficient confidence in yourself. Look for people and situations that will encourage you and support you in your endeavor.

The following formula has always been helpful to me when confronting obstacles.

1. Observe yourself without judgment.
2. Tell the truth about what is happening.
3. Accept things as they are.

4. Remember your goal.
5. Get back on the path as soon as possible.

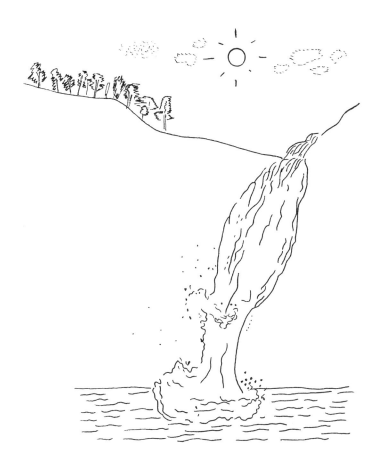

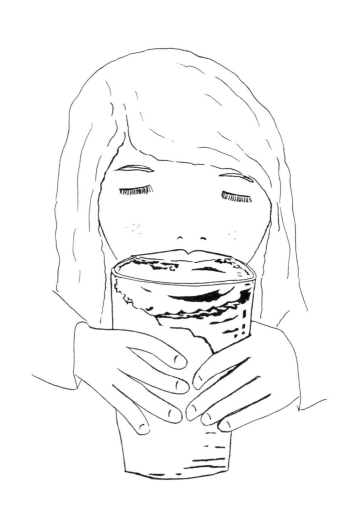

Fasting for Health

YOUR MIND, WHICH DETERMINES your moods and behavior, is influenced by the condition of your blood. To purify your mind, you need to purify your blood. There are two types of poisons in your blood. One is *physical*, such as unclean food, air, water and drugs. The other is *spiritual*, such as unclean thoughts and feelings.

Through the blood you inherit from your parents and ancestors not only their physical weaknesses but also their mental make-up. These remain as memories in your blood. Another way you pollute your blood is by eating animals which have impure blood from ingesting chemicals, hormones and the like. You are also taking into your body their nature and their fears.

Even after years on a vegetarian diet I still felt tired on occasion, so I began doing short fasts, one to three weeks at a time, along with enemas twice a day. When I saw the filth which came out of my body, it became clear why I was feeling so tired. After each fast I felt stronger and more enthusiastic, so I continued this practice.

When you fast you actually give your body a chance to rest, cleanse and heal itself. Fasting does not have to be difficult, though you might feel some physical discomfort at times. A positive attitude and an understanding of what your body is experiencing will be very helpful. Fasting is not starving. (The only creatures that you starve are your worms.) Any discipline you take upon yourself by your own choice with the intention to better yourself does not cause suffering. You can actually look forward to feeling better than you usually do.

The following programs are great preparations for a week or more of **total fasting**. Any one of them can be considered a type of fast, as the body may go through a cleansing period similar to that experienced while on a total fast.

1. For those who still eat meat, fish, eggs and dairy products— give these up for a month and eat natural rice, soy products, beans, legumes, cereals, and vegetables, fruits and nuts.

2. For those who have been on a vegetarian diet for a while—go on a diet of raw vegetables, fruits and nuts for a month.
3. For those already eating raw food exclusively—go on fresh juices from either fruits or vegetables, or eat only fruit for a month.

A fasting program for a week or more

Necessary

- Mineral water or water which has been **purified.**
- Keep away from negative people; try to be silent as much as possible.
- Go for walks in nature. It is good to be around trees or running water.
- Sleep in a clean room with windows open; if you are cold, use a cover. Fresh air is a must.
- If you feel weak or sick, take an enema and rest in the air.

Good

- Get full body massage.
- First thing in the morning, drink **Ginseng tea plus honey** or diluted **wheat-grass juice** or **wheat grass tablets.** (Pines) Then take an

enema with camomile tea or **wheat grass powder** or **garlic powder** (mixed in luke warm **purified** water).

- During the day drink **lemonade** made from fresh lemons and pure water with organic uncooked **honey**, which contains bee pollen and propolis or drink brewed **parsley** with some rosemary.
- A tablespoon of **Psyllium husk** drunk in a glass of water, morning and night, enables mucus and old, sticky feces to come out more easily. (Psyllium can be purchased in health food stores.)
- Herb tea of a laxative nature. (I prefer Super Dieters Tea from Laci Le Beau.)
- Before showering, brush entire body with **natural bristle brush.** This gets rid of dead cells and will revitalize and increase the eliminative capacity of your skin.
- Shower at least twice a day. Follow each hot shower with cold water. This too has a rejuvenating effect.
- **Sauna** or **steam** room once a week.
- Exercise: **Yoga postures** or any other daily exercise.
- **Breathing exercise:** at least 30 deep breaths a day.
- Change clothing after every shower or bath. Check your sheets and towels for a bad odor or stain.

Optional

- Write down your thoughts, dreams and realizations. Keep a journal. (You'll find that you will have many new revelations during fasts.)
- Before sleep, take an enema with **camomile tea** or with wheat grass powder or garlic powder.
- Before sleep, rub stomach with **castor oil,** then cover it with a hot water bottle wrapped in a towel. (This helps loosen old crust from colon walls.)
- Sit or lie in indirect sunlight and in the fresh air with a minimum of clothing for an hour daily.
- Take rejuvenating herbs which assist cleansing, healing and rebuilding of the body. (Sunrider has an excellent selection.)

It is known that all the organs of the body are affected by the condition of the colon, so it is necessary to cleanse it through proper foods, short fasts, and having enemas whenever necessary. But even after the colon becomes clean it will not return to its original shape unless you maintain a steady and consistent **raw food** diet for a period of one to seven years, depending on your age and the condition of your colon.

Here are some benefits you can expect from fasting for one week or more:

- Deeper meditations.
- Deeper, quieter sleep.
- Regular and easy bowel movements.
- Disappearance of many fears and childhood traumas.
- More peace and love.
- More enthusiasm for life.
- More patience with self and others.
- Less hunger and less food required. Craving foods which are natural.
- Disappearance of destructive habits, both mental and physical.

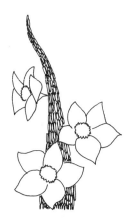

Fasting with Enemas

During a fast the body automatically starts "house cleaning." All the filth and toxic wastes which have accumulated in the tissues for years, causing disease and premature aging, are loosened and expelled from the system. The alimentary canal, the digestive and the eliminative systems are the main roads by which these toxins are thrown out of the body. Enemas during fasting greatly assist the body in its cleansing effort by washing out all toxic wastes. If you don't get rid of this waste as soon as possible, it will be absorbed back into the bloodstream and could cause nausea, dizziness and fainting. This is what I experienced when I wouldn't do enemas. During my last fasts I did not suffer any discomfort because I did enemas whenever I felt the need. Another good reason to do enemas is that it helps usher out the many worms that live in the colon.

In most fasting clinics in Europe they give enemas twice a day and colonics at least once a week.

Right posture for an enema will enable the water to reach far into the colon. The water should be luke-warm mixed with either camomile tea or wheat grass powder or garlic powder. For lubricating the rectum, I use Crisco.

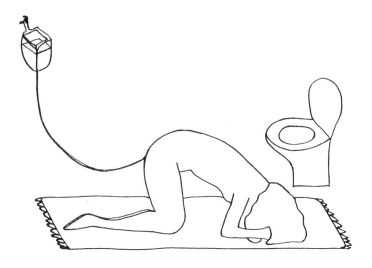

Either **wheat grass** or **garlic powder** will help in destroying and expelling worms and the rebuilding of important intestinal bacteria which aid in the digestion of food.

An enema bag or feminine hygiene bag can be purchased at any drugstore.

It is virtually impossible to become completely healthy if the colon is not clean of old feces and does not function perfectly. As you will see in the following drawing, there are points directly connected to specific organs throughout the colon. For example, if point 27 is blocked by old feces or the colon is twisted or distorted in this area there will be problems with eyesight. And the same goes for all other centers and organs of the body.

Throughout its entire length, the colon extracts nutrients from the food which comes to it from the small intestine. In addition, it is the function of the ascending colon to gather from the glands in its walls the intestinal flora needed to lubricate the colon. But if the colon is coated with fecal incrustation, the glands will not produce the necessary intestinal flora for lubrication. Lack of lubrication only intensifies the state of constipation and generates toxemia. Pimples are usually the first indication of it.

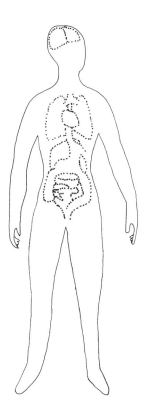

In the following diagram I mention only the most important points in the colon. A more detailed diagram can be found in Dr. Norman W. Walker's book, *Colon Health.* (Both diagrams here are reprinted with permission of Norwalk Press, Prescott, AZ 96301.)

Points in the colon which directly influence the various centers and organs in the body.

1	Region of worms	16	Testes
2	Pituitary gland	17	Bladder
3	Thymus gland	18	Prostate
4	Nasal catarrh	19	Uterus
5	Mammary glands	20	Genital glands
6	Thyroid gland	21	Mammary glands
7	Liver	22	Throat
8	Gall bladder	23	Bronchials
9	Heart	24	Esophagus
10	Pylorus	25	Trachea
11	Stomach	26	Adenoids
12	Pancreas	27	Eyes
13	Adrenal glands	28	Tonsils
14	Kidneys	29	Ears
15	Genital glands	30	End of small intestines

This drawing represents a healthy, natural colon of a baby.

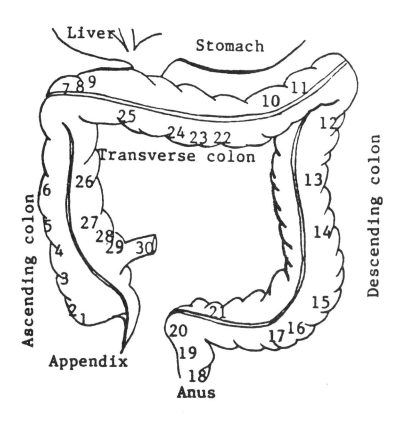

From an x-ray of a distorted colon of a 36-year-old woman who ate meat and drank alcoholic beverages.

The cut in the ascending colon shows the crust of 20-year-old feces. The new feces must pass through the tiny space in the middle.

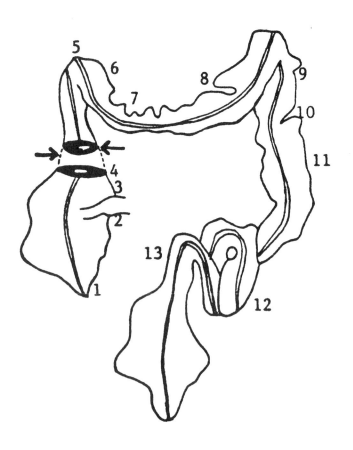

Her problems were:

1 Tape worm
2 Sinus
3 Trouble with vision
4 Indigestion
5 Enlargement of liver
6 Heart trouble
7 Low blood pressure

Disturbances of:
8 Stomach
9 Pancreas
10 Adrenals
11 Kidneys
12 Bladder
13 Menstruation

One of the main reasons we feel a constant desire to eat is because our body does not receive the proper nutrients it should derive from food as it approaches our colon. If the vessels through which the body receives its nutrients are clogged up, the body is not fed, no matter how much we eat. These vessels get clogged from the consumption of large amounts of meat, starch and refined foods which have a tendency to stick to the walls of the colon and form a plaster-like coating which interferes with the process of proper assimilation and elimination. If we want to correct this condition, it is necessary to change our eating habits to include much more "wet food" (fruits and vegetables).

The colon, which has the important function of body eliminations, is distorted and cannot function properly as a result of eating the wrong foods, lack of exercise and suppressed emotions. The result is constipation. Nearly every person who grew up on the "normal" diet of Western civilization is constipated, whether he evacuates daily or not.

You cannot reach perfect health so long as your sewage system—your colon—is clogged with putrefied feces and toxic wastes.

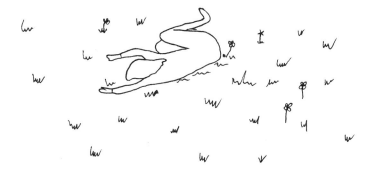

Conscious Breathing

USUALLY THE ONLY TIME we are conscious of our breath is when we sit still to meditate or during vigorous exercise. The breath is our connection to our soul and spirit. Through the breath you receive your most important food. Without breathing you stop living in your physical body. Your breath should be free and easy and constant. If it becomes heavy and shallow, it is a sign of aging and tension in the body.

The breath is obstructed for several reasons:

1. Not enough physical exercise
2. Wrong foods and quantities
3. Stress and emotional problems

To remedy this you can start by observing the rhythm of your breath while sitting still, then while walking. Observing the breath while eating will give you an indication of whether you are eating the right foods or too much food. Then, observe the breath when you are emotionally upset. Notice that you are holding your breath, which causes more tension.

Get into the habit of always observing your breath in the navel area. This is a good habit to develop. It will eventually give you power over your life.

Right Rest

When your breathing is full and rhythmic, when you feel no heaviness or difficulty in breathing, then your body is receiving the right amount of oxygen and you feel peaceful.

Following is an exercise in relaxation designed to improve your breathing. It can be done in a sitting or a lying position. It is best done in a clean and quiet place where you will not be disturbed.

You can record yourself speaking slowly and softly with relaxing music in the background. Listen to it when you have about ten minutes to relax. You will find that hearing your own voice can be very soothing. You will benefit from this exercise even by reading it to yourself.

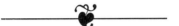

A Relaxation Exercise

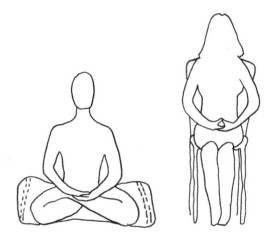

SIT OR LIE DOWN ON YOUR BACK, giving all your weight to the floor. Place your arms beside your body and close your eyes. Leave your mouth slightly open and breathe through your nose. Breathe well; observe your breathing.

Continue to observe your breathing but this time start to breathe a little deeper than you usually do. Continue to breathe deeply. Notice how with each breath you become more relaxed and more at ease.

Breathe deeply; feel your legs breathing. From your toes all the way up to the end of your thighs, your legs are breathing and relaxing; your legs are breathing and relaxing. . . . Good.

Breathe deeply; feel your torso breathing. From your upper thighs all the way up to your shoulders, your torso is breathing and relaxing, your torso is breathing and relaxing.

Breathe deeply; feel your arms breathing. From your shoulders down to your finger tips, your arms are breathing and relaxing; your arms are breathing and relaxing.

Breathe deeply; feel your neck and head breathing and relaxing, your neck and head breathing and relaxing. . . . Good.

Breathe deeply; feel your face breathing. From your chin up to your forehead, your entire face is breathing and relaxing, your entire face is breathing and relaxing. . . . Good.

Now breathe, and feel your entire body breathing and relaxing. Your whole body is breathing and relaxing. Every atom is vibrating with life. Breathe and feel every cell of your body breathing and being renewed. . . . Good.

Breathe, and feel every organ of your body being replenished and cleansed. Breathe and feel the peace in your body as you breathe.

Breathe, and feel your body revitalizing as you breathe. The more you breathe the better you feel; the more you breathe, the more relaxed you become.

Now, go back to your regular way of breathing. Let the body breathe the way it wants to. Don't interfere with the natural breath flow, just observe the breathing. . . . Good.

Breathe, and let the breath flow easily and freely throughout your body, completely and totally revitalizing your whole body.

Breathe, and know that your brain and all the organs in your body are replenished, cleansed and renewed. Stay connected to the breathing, feel the breath in your navel area. . . . Good.

Now, stretch your arms over your head, stretch your legs, open your mouth wide and yawn, and . . . relax.

Breathe, and notice the way you feel inside your body now. Notice how your body is. Continue to observe your breathing.

Now your mind and body are totally cleansed from all impurities. Your blood is flowing freely throughout your body. You feel refreshed, awake and fully concentrated. You feel alive. You feel good inside your body now.

Breathe, and remember that if ever you feel lost or tense, you will be able to return to this peaceful state simply by reestablishing your connection with your breath.

Breathe, and feel your breath flowing in your navel. Whenever you feel ready to open your eyes you will do so easily, and you will continue to feel wonderful with your eyes open. Your breath will flow easily and freely and you will stay conscious of your breath flowing in your navel. Be at peace . . . .

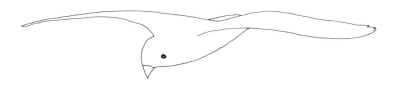

Five Great Exercises

YOUR BODY IS A FINE INSTRUMENT. Just as a musical instrument cannot be played properly when it is out of tune, so your body, which is your most vital instrument, cannot serve you properly when too tense or too loose.

The following five exercises will tune your body and give you balance and energy all day. They should be done first thing in the morning, before meditation, before eating, and before you start your day.

Repeat each exercise at least twice. Do them to rhythmic music, in an easy manner with attention to the breath flow.

Before you start lie down on your back, giving all your weight to the floor, and just observe your breath flow. Once you have come to a steady, rhythmic breath, you can begin your first exercise.

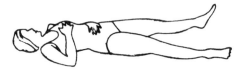

I
1. Press knees to chest and release.
2. Roll backwards and forwards.
3. Move knees from right to left.
4. Rest flat on your back; breathe well.

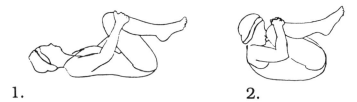

1.   2.

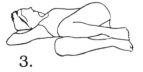
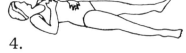

3.   4.

II

1. Bring your legs up, hands supporting your back, chin touching your chest.
2. Let one leg down over your head, change legs.
3. Bring both legs down. Rest and breathe well.
4. Bend knees so they touch your ears.
5. Hold onto your toes and roll back and forth.
6. Lie flat on your back. Observe your breathing in the navel area.

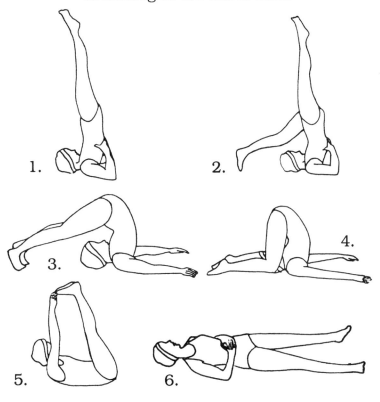

III

1. Sit down on the floor, left leg straight at a 45° angle, right foot bent against the left thigh. Hold onto your left foot with both hands, bring your forehead to your left knee, or as close to it as possible, for four breaths. Bring left ear to knee for four breaths. Bring forehead to knee for four breaths. Bring right ear to knee for four breaths. Do this several times with attention on the breathing.

2. Change legs and do the same movements towards the right leg. Change again.

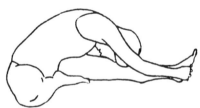

1.

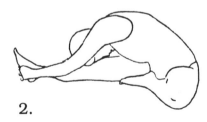

2.

IV

1. Stand up straight, knees touching, feet parallel.
2. Send right leg back, keep it straight. Bend left leg.
3. Raise both arms up over your head.
4. Bring arms down.
5. Bring right leg forward and start again, this time sending left leg back.

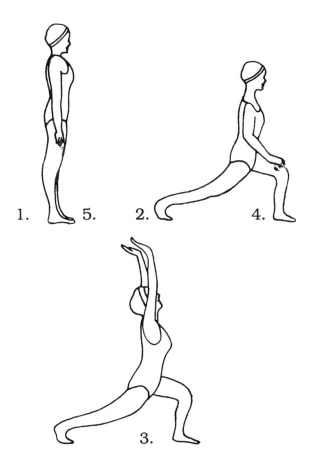

1.   5.   2.   4.

3.

V

1. Legs are open wide, feet parallel. Lock your fingers behind your back, pulling shoulders and head back.

2. Look up and start moving forward until your back is parallel to the floor.

3. Move to your right looking far to the right. Move left, looking far to the left. Come back to center.

4. Let your arms fall over your head while fingers are still locked. Look between your legs. Move your forehead to right knee and then to left knee. Come back to center and bend your knees. Move from right to left.

5. Straighten your legs, pull your arms, shoulders and head back and slowly move back to a standing position. Release your arms. Shake both arms and legs and repeat.

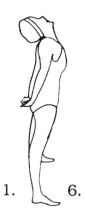

1.   6.

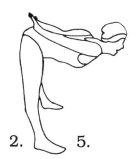

2.   5.

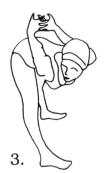

3.

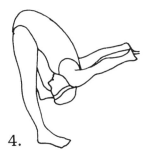

4.

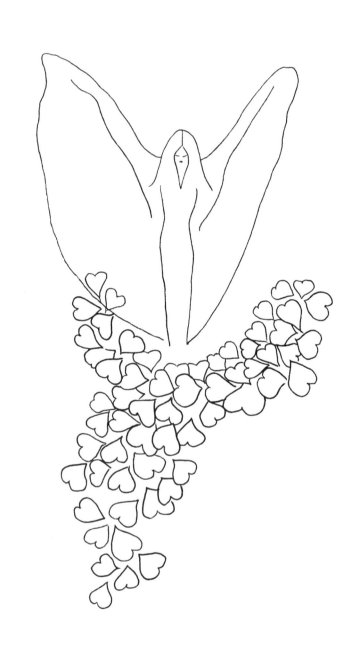

Perfect Health

PERFECT HEALTH IN BODY AND MIND is the prerequisite for spiritual evolution and for raising your vibration.

It may seem an impossibility to some of you who feel sick or too old to start the repair work. But I assure you, no matter what your present condition, you can reach near perfect health in just a few years and have a peaceful, productive life for as long as you choose.

Perhaps you don't even know how a perfectly healthy person looks or how he feels and behaves. For this reason I have outlined some of those attributes for you.

A PERFECTLY HEALTHY PERSON IS:

- Fearless.
- Sensitive.
- Energetic.
- Balanced.
- Enthusiastic.
- Happy and loving.
- Peaceful and calm.

A PERFECTLY HEALTHY PERSON CAN:

- Concentrate and memorize easily.
- Respond peacefully and calmly in every situation.
- Speak little and clearly.
- Sleep little and quietly, and wake up at sunrise alert.
- Be satisfied with small and simple meals.
- Not create accidents or any other misfortunes.
- Accomplish things thoroughly and with ease.
- Have a calming influence over those around him.
- Be attentive to his breath.
- Be aware of the workings of his body.

PERFECT HEALTH

In Vilcabamba Valley in Ecuador there are people who live over 120 years. Their diet is mainly vegetarian, favoring oranges, bananas and apples. They eat only an ounce of meat a week and no animal fat. They work until the end of their lives.

The ancient Greeks, before Lycurgus, knew of generations that reached the age of 200 years. The Pelasgians favored apples. They were able to race and win against their horses. Throughout their lives they stayed tall and kept their natural hair color.

The Hunza people near India maintained perfect health and youthfulness throughout their lives. They had no need for doctors, as they never got sick. They ate mostly fruit only once a day.

Professor Hilton Hotema, himself over 90 years of age, thoroughly investigated the topic of longevity. He found the following essentials for a long life:

- High altitude mountains, preferably in tropical areas.
- A fruitarian diet.
- Little sex activity.
- Pollution free air.
- Loving friends.
- Fasting.

Earlier it was mentioned that energy is lost through:

- Improper use of the body.
- Improper use of the mind.
- Improper use of the spirit.

We now know that energy can be acquired and accumulated through the proper use of body, mind and spirit. Just as it took time and effort to pollute our bodies and minds, it will take time and effort to cleanse them.

One of the ways I used to clean my thoughts was by writing affirmations exactly opposite to what I was thinking. No matter what negative thought would come into my mind, I would take my notebook and write the opposite. Soon, I started to get great results. What I wrote became so.

The following affirmations are **my ten commandments.** Every one of them is essential to maintaining harmony in body, mind and heart. You might want to use these or write your own.

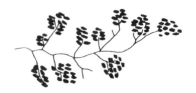

Ten Commandments for Perfect Health

1. I breathe consciously, fully and freely.

2. I love truth. I am always truthful.

3. I agree only to what I intend to do. I joyfully keep all my agreements.

4. I do all that is necessary to improve myself. I support others who contribute to the quality of life.

5. My positive power is stronger than any negative force.

6. I love people unconditionally.
   I forgive everyone who hurts me.

7. I am complete and whole. All
   knowledge and power are within me.

8. I am free of my past. I live in the
   present. I welcome the changes in
   my life.

9. I do all that is necessary to keep
   my body in perfect health.

10. I do not harm or destroy any life.

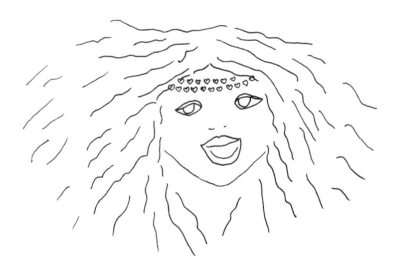

Thanks to God

How do I feel?
Every day I feel more love
Everyone feels my love
My life is flowing
I am growing
Thanks to God!

What's happening?
Things happen as they should
Always for my good
I am happy and clear
More positive each year
Thanks to God!

What am I doing?
My duties I fulfill
I receive what I will
From mistakes I learn
From every loss I gain
Thanks to God!

What's in the future?
I have all I need
My life is at ease
I look forward
To more peace
As I sow so I reap
Thanks to God!

Books of Interest

THIS LIST IS ONLY A FRACTION of all the great books I have read. Though I mention only one book by each author, all the books written by the following authors were inspiring and informative.

FOR THE BODY

AIROLA, PAAVO. Dr. *How to Get Well.* Health Plus, 1974.

EHRET, ARNOLD. *Mucusless Diet Healing System.* Ehret Literature Publishing Co., 1972.

GRAY, ROBERT. *The Colon Health Handbook.* Rockridge Publishing Co., 1980.

ROBBINS, JOHN. *Diet for a New America.* Stillpoint Publishing, 1987.

SZEKELY, E. B. *The Essene Gospel of Peace.* I.B.S. International, 1978.

WALKER, N. W., Dr. *Become Younger.* Norwalk Press, 1978.

YESUDIAN, S. & HAICH, E. *Yoga and Health.* New York: Harper Brothers, 1953.

FOR THE MIND

EMERY, STEWART. *Actualizations.* Doubleday & Co., 1977.

FULLER, R.B. *Critical Path.* St. Martin's Press, 1981.

KEYES, JR., KEN. *Handbook to Higher Consciousness.* Living Love Center, 1975.

OUSPENSKY, P. D. *In Search of the Miraculous.* Routledge & Kegan Paul, 1950.

PERCIVAL, H. W. *Man and Woman and Child.* The Word Foundation, 1979.

RAJNEESH, BHAGWAN SHREE. *The Book of the Secrets.* Harper & Row, 1977.

FOR THE HEART

BENNETT, J. G. *Long Pilgrimage.* Hodder & Stoughton, 1965.

EASWARAN, E. *Gandhi the Man.* Nilgiri Press, 1978.

HAICH, ELISABETH. *Initiation.* Seed Center, 1974.

LEVI. *The Aquarian Gospel of Jesus the Christ.* DeVorss & Co., 1972.

RAMALA CENTRE. *The Revelation of Ramala.* Neville Spearman (Jersey) Ltd., 1978.

SAI BABA, SATHYA. *Voice of the Avatar.* M. Gulab Singh & Sons, 1980.

SIVANANDA, SRI SWAMI. *Spiritual Experiences.* The Divine Life Society, 1957, 1986.

TWEEDIE, IRINA. *Daughter of Fire.* Blue Dolphin Publishing, Inc., 1986.

YOGANANDA, PARAMHANSA. *The Autobiography of a Yogi.* Self-Realization Fellowship, 1946.

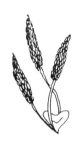

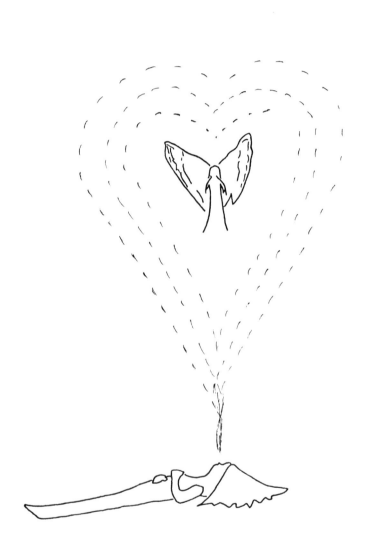

OTHER BOOKS from

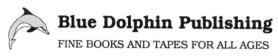

Blue Dolphin Publishing

FINE BOOKS AND TAPES FOR ALL AGES

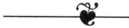

Are You Really Too Sensitive?	
Marcy Calhoun	$12.95
Blatant Raw Foodist Propaganda	
Joe Alexander	$12.95
The Butterfly Rises Kit Tremaine	$12.95
Coming to Life James L. Doak	$9.95
Daughter of Fire Irina Tweedie	$19.95
Do Less . . . and Be Loved More	
Peg Tompkins	$8.95
I Need Help! A Stroke Victim's Plea	
Helen Underwood	$8.95
Mary's Message to the World	
Annie Kirkwood	$12.95
A Practical Guide to Creative Senility	
Donovan Bess	$9.95
Points: Improve Your Self-Image	
Dave Gustafson	$12.95
Tastes of Tuscany Liana Figone	$19.95
Turning to the Source Dhiravamsa	$19.95

Write for free catalog or order directly from
Blue Dolphin Publishing
P.O. Box 1908, Nevada City, CA 95959
(916) 265-6923

N OGAH LORD HAS STUDIED AND TAUGHT in America, India, and Israel for the past twenty years. She gives lectures and conducts seminars on Living in Harmony.

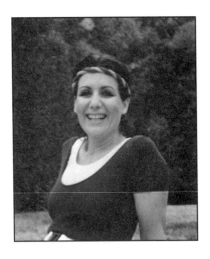

For further information, please contact:
Nogah Lord, P.O. Box 4073
Lynchburg, VA 24502